Table of Cont‹

CW00401377

Forward by Author

"As a practicing healthcare provider, I diagnose, treat and prescribe medicine for my patients every day. We work together as a team: MD, DO, PA NP and NDs. We have confidence in our methodology and the algorithm for treatment. We help people. It is a rewarding practice beyond belief.

As a well-rounded human being who is constantly striving to grow and improve personally and professionally, I like to think it's important to step back and see the big picture, too. There is much more out there than pharmaceutical medicines to treat our ailments. Our modern medicine system is heavily reliant on pharmaceuticals. I think it is important we have perspective to realize the multitude of ways to treat a human being – treat the whole person, which includes the mental, physical and spiritual aspects of one's health. It is the art of medicine. That is why I am excited to be doing what I do."

Why I Wrote this eBook

Most people don't know what Metabolic Syndrome is. I'd like to help increase that awareness, because it is a growing problem. 1 out of 3 Americans have Metabolic Syndrome (aka Syndrome X). The statistic increase to a dramatic 50% of those over age 60 who have Metabolic Syndrome[1].

It is a cluster of risk factors, including increased blood sugar, increased waist circumference, abnormal cholesterol and elevated blood pressure. Even meeting 3 of these parameters qualifies metabolic syndrome.
Those with Metabolic Syndrome are at increased risk for heart disease and stroke.
Lifestyle changes can potentially reverse this diagnosis.

Diabetes runs in my family, so I have tried to keep this in the forefront of my thinking. Despite eating healthy and exercising after having our baby, I developed what I believe was a form of Metabolic Syndrome. It's almost as if my body tried to hold on to every last pound, despite my best efforts. A lot of people attribute this to aging, 'Oh, it's just part of getting older.' But through my research, I now understand even more about this metabolic dysfunction at the cellular and mitochondrial level.

Learning more in depth about metabolic function on a cellular level has been intriguing. For instance, studies link optimized metabolism with decreased risk of cancer and increased longevity. Not just a longer life, but better quality of life. The stuff that really matters.

Anyway, this is a long-winded way of saying, I'm really passionate about this. In part, that is what motivated me to develop a natural product to assist in metabolic dysfunction. I am excited to share my knowledge and guidance in this process, and I'm hopeful that you are willing to share the wealth of knowledge, too!

Cheers to living a better life,
Jessie

What Is Metabolic Syndrome?

Metabolic Syndrome (otherwise known as Syndrome X) is the co-occurrence of certain risk factors, which increase susceptibility for Type 2 Diabetes and cardiovascular disease. The risk factors include: increased waist circumference or belly fat, high blood sugar levels, high triglycerides, elevated blood pressure, and a low HDL (good) cholesterol level. Meeting even 3 of these criteria, qualifies Metabolic Syndrome.[1,2*]

Criteria:
Answering 'yes' to 3 of the 5 questions:

- Is your waist circumference ≥ 88 cm (women)
  or ≥ 102 cm (men)?
  [inches: ≥ 35 in. (women) or ≥ 40 in. (men)]
- Are your fasting blood sugar levels ≥ 100
  (or have you been diagnosed with diabetes?)
- Is your HDL (good) cholesterol level ≤ 50 (women)
  or ≤ 40 (men)?
- Are your triglycerides ≥ 150 (men or women)
  (or are you on medicine for cholesterol?)
- Do you have elevated blood pressure ≥ 130/85
  (or are you on medicine for blood pressure?)

Do you meet any 3 of the 5 bullet points?

If so, welcome to the Metabolic Syndrome Club.

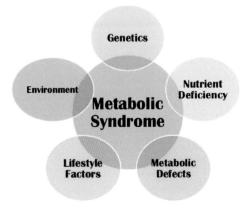

ee Table 1 in Appendix for a breakdown of the universally accepted criteria for Metabolic Syndrome)

nk of it as a continuum: **Metabolic Syndrome → Pre-Diabetes →   Type 2 Diabetes**

What Causes Metabolic Syndrome?

Metabolic Syndrome is a complex disorder that is often multi-factorial. It can involve a genetic predisposition, but there is strong association linking environmental and dietary impacts. (To be noted: there may also be an overlay of other conditions such as: PCOS [polycystic ovarian syndrome], OSA [obstructive sleep apnea], thyroid disorder, or hormonal changes [i.e. association with pregnancy and the postpartum period] linked with metabolic disorder.) The genes related to metabolic syndrome can be inherited, but in fact the great majority of causation often boils down to lifestyle choices.

Simply put, lifestyle choices in this context pertain to over-eating and a routinely sedentary lifestyle. The human body responds to chronic high-caloric malnutrition via fat deposition. High-caloric malnutrition results from a combination of *excess calories* along with *poor quality types of food* consumed.

Eating too many calories in a day leads to the storage of fat molecules in adipose tissue cells. Adipose (fat) tissue – and specifically visceral adipose tissue – has been found to have a direct correlation with insulin resistance. Visceral adiposity means the presence of a high degree of fatty tissue within the abdomen. That is why 'waist circumference' is the first qualifying factor above. Visceral adipose tissue causes a cascade of pro-inflammatory markers, which itself is implicated in insulin resistance and is associated with cardiovascular disease[2]. Portion sizes are important to remember when it comes to calorie intake.

Standard USDA recommendations: ≤ 2,000 calories per day.

Generally speaking, consistently eating more than 2,000 calories in a day will typically lead to adipose deposition and weight gain, unless you are extremely active to off-set this. Each person has a basal metabolic rate (BMR). Lean muscle mass tends to increase your BMR, which means, people who incorporate weight lifting tend to burn more calories at rest than those without as much muscle mass. Calorie-restriction generally leads to a decrease in adipose tissue and resultant weight loss, so the goal would be to consume closer to ~1200-1600 calories per day (caloric deficit), if you are trying to lose fat.

Aside from calories, the quality of food matters, too. Heavy consumption of poor-quality food, such as refined/processed food, converts into sugar very quickly in the bloodstream, and can trigger a cascade of inflammation. These types of highly refined, poor-quality food often don't contain enough nutrients such as protein, vitamins, trace elements, and fiber to nourish your body or support a healthy metabolism. Habitual high intake of processed and refined carbohydrates contributes to insulin resistance and has been linked to weight gain and obesity.

Hence, both **quality** and **quantity** of food intake matters.

In this book, we will discuss tried and true solutions, including diet and exercise. We will get into the nitty gritty of this. We will also discuss certain prescription medications and natural dietary supplements, like our product BestFormin that can help combat Metabolic Syndrome.

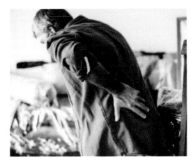

1. Fatigue, brain fogginess or inability to focus can indicate metabolic dysfunction.

2. Excessive thirst, sweet-smelling breath and frequent urination can be signs of high blood sugar.

3. Intestinal bloating – *some* intestinal gas is produced from carbohydrates that humans cannot digest and absorb; consider for instance, gluten sensitivity or intolerance.

4. Excess sleepiness, especially after meals due to blood sugar crash.

5. Weight gain, fat storage, difficulty losing weight – for most people, excess weight is from high fat storage; the fat is generally stored in and around abdominal organs in both males and females. It is currently suspected that hormones produced in that fatty adipose tissue are a precipitating cause of insulin resistance.

6. Headaches can sometimes be caused by increased blood pressure. Insulin contributes to the body's vasculature response, and hence plays a role in blood pressure regulation.

7. Psychological effects, including depression, can be related to the metabolism disorder resulting from insulin resistance.

8. Increased hunger/cravings/insatiable appetite. Due to insulin resistance, your body doesn't recognize that it is getting enough sugar. Even though there is plenty of sugar in the bloodstream, it can't get inside the cells adequately because of the resistance to insulin.

• • •

Now that we've addressed the definition, cause and symptoms of Metabolic Syndrome, let's take a step back and ensure we understand how the body breaks down and processes the food that you put into your body.

Your Body's Functioning 101

•Your body needs energy to function. You eat a meal.

•Your body breaks that meal down into: 1) fats, 2) proteins, and 3) carbohydrates, and ultimately turns each of them into ATP molecules of energy.

•Carbs are the most immediate source of energy, which get broken down into glucose (sugar) fastest.

•Glucose needs to get into your cells, to function properly, and get converted into ATP for energy.

•If glucose cannot efficiently get inside the cells, that leaves one with 'high blood sugar levels'.

•Insulin acts like a key to allow glucose to get inside your cells. ➡️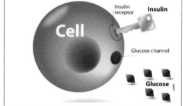

•Those with metabolic syndrome, pre-diabetes or type 2 diabetes, often have some degree of 'insulin resistance': the pancreas secretes insulin, but the cells are resistant to it. *(Why? Visceral adiposity.)*

•This can confuse the body's regulatory feedback system because the cells don't detect that they are getting enough glucose on the inside. As a result, the body up-regulates the process to make even MORE sugar available in your blood (via mechanisms like breaking down glycogen, the storage form of glucose from your liver, to make glucose more bio-available)...even though it doesn't need any more sugar!

•Clearly this is a dysfunctional cycle that needs to get addressed; otherwise the process continues until the body stores excess fat molecules, you have increased fat deposits and can develop type 2 diabetes.

How do you stop the cycle?

•Activating the protein enzyme in cells called 'AMPK' is one way to help fix this dysfunctional cycle.

•AMPK is the master metabolic switch for your cells.
   -An enzyme we all have; it initiates intracellular signals that bring glucose inside the cell where it needs to be to function properly (despite any insulin resistance).
   -It by-passes the dysfunctional cycle and gets the glucose inside the cells via a different intracellular transport system.

•You can activate AMPK via: <u>vigorous exercise</u>, <u>calorie-restricted diet</u> or <u>intermittent periods of fasting</u>.
   -During exercise, activated AMPK increases glucose uptake and fatty acid oxidation.
   -This tells your body to bring in and utilize the glucose as energy.
   -It also supports mitochondrial activity: important to keep metabolism high and fuel your muscles.

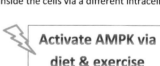

BOTTOM LINE: To break the viscous cycle of storing fat, it is important to have a healthy diet, with regular exercise in order to help activate AMPK. We will be talking about other natural ways to activate AMPK – more to come.

What Can I Do to Help Reverse Metabolic Syndrome?

I'm so glad you asked. Metabolic Syndrome can be improved and perhaps even reversed in time. Since your body fat percentage has a corresponding relationship with insulin, as you drop fat and weight (especially in midsection and torso) your body will gradually improve insulin sensitivity. Please, read on.

Diet

Overall, it is important to eat a well-balanced diet that tends to mimic purity. If I had to make a comparison to what an ideal diet would look like, you'd have two options: 1) Think Caveman (Paleo) or 2) Mediterranean diet.

That being said, please understand that the word 'diet' in this circumstance indicates that of a paradigm shift. It refers to a lifestyle change with the purpose being to make more good choices than the bad ones. The word 'diet' here, does not mean something you do for a few weeks to lose weight. It does not mean something you guilt yourself over, depriving yourself of (occasional) cravings, resulting in over-indulging later.

⭐ If you are to take any main message home after reading the section on Diet here, please <u>let it be this</u>: Focus on your goals. Focus on eating well-rounded, nutritious meals. Forgive and love yourself. Don't punish yourself. If you have a craving, it's ok to occasionally indulge with a *reasonable* portion size. Just try to make more good than bad decisions, consistently. Set daily, weekly and monthly goals. Hold yourself accountable.

Nutritional Recommendations

Vegetables: No need to limit vegetables. Eat as many vegetables as you'd like. Try vegetables you've never eaten before. You may be surprised. Try to substitute vegetables as side dishes when you can. *EXTRA CREDIT:* kale, spinach, beets, broccoli, Brussels sprouts, carrots, eggplant, zucchini, bell peppers, avocado (some people consider avocado a fruit, but we'll leave it here for now)

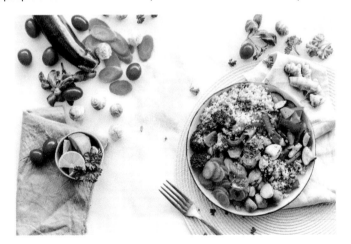

Protein: Optimize your protein intake. Protein is important in your diet. Proteins get broken down into amino acids – the 'building blocks of life', crucial for cellular function, structure and regeneration.

We honor your culinary preference, whether that be pescatarian, vegetarian, vegan or omnivore. In accordance with your respective dietary preference, we encourage protein. If you eat meat, we encourage you to focus on lean meats. Chicken, poultry, fish. If you are a vegetarian, complementary proteins such as beans and (brown) rice are good. Nuts and legumes, i.e. black beans, lentil beans and chickpeas are excellent sources of protein. Eggs, shellfish and peanuts, peanut butter, almond butter (if no nut allergy). Whey protein, soybean or tofu. Almonds are a healthy source of protein and incorporate the healthy, good type of fat in your diet. Minimize red meats since overconsumption of these can be correlated with heart disease.

EXTRA CREDIT: salmon is an excellent source of protein; it also contains essential Omega-3 fatty acids, which help lower your triglycerides and are heart-healthy. Try to incorporate salmon into your diet once per week.

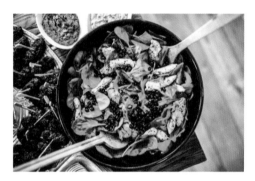

Grains: Focus on whole grain if you choose to incorporate grains. Brown rice, whole wheat pasta, whole grain couscous, whole wheat bread… high fiber is the key. Oats are also an excellent type of grain, which actually help to improve cholesterol.

Your body takes longer to break down high fiber. This results in you feeling fuller for longer. It also utilizes more energy for your body to break down these 'complex carbohydrates', which means you expend more energy metabolizing whole grain. (It also means there is a more gradual release of insulin into your blood stream, not a spike in blood sugar that you'd get with eating highly processed, refined foods like white bread, white rice or plain pasta.) *Tip: organic brown rice in grocery's frozen section!

EXTRA CREDIT: superfoods in this category include chia seeds, flaxseed, quinoa or amaranth.

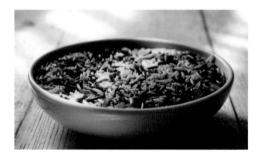

ruits: Allow fruits in moderation because they can sometimes spike blood sugar. Fruit tends to be a
reat source of fiber and also a good way to curb your sweet-tooth in a healthier way than sugar-
ortified, processed foods. Diversify your fruit intake because different fruits have varying health
enefits.
XTRA CREDIT: superfoods such as blueberries, raspberries, blackberries, açai berry, cranberry,
omegranate and dragon fruit include good antioxidants.

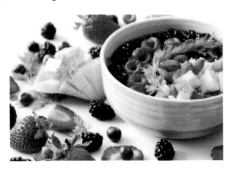

ts: Since there are such things as 'good' and 'bad' fats, maximize the good and minimize the bad.
ood fats would include things like: olive oil, avocados, almonds/nuts, chia seed, flax seed, dark
ocolate, egg, salmon.
ese types of 'good' fats lead to feeling satiated (full) for longer and actually can increase your HDL*
ood) cholesterol, which is heart-protective. Choose organic butter over margarine.
inimize intake of the 'bad' fats: margarine, trans fats, saturated fats, canola or hydrogenated oil.
minate fried/deep fried food.
t in the habit of checking nutrition labels. Avoid anything that has Trans fat, and try to minimize the
ount of saturated fat.
TRA CREDIT: grass-fed butter is a better choice due to intrinsic Omega 3, 6 and 9. As above-
entioned, aim for including mostly good fats in your diet: olive oil, avocados, almonds/nuts, chia seed,
xseed, dark chocolate, egg, salmon.

*de note: HDL stands for high-density lipoprotein, and it is known as the good cholesterol because it
ps remove other forms of cholesterol from your bloodstream. Higher levels of HDL cholesterol are
own to be 'cardio-protective' because they actually lower the risk of heart disease.
ontrast, LDL stands for low-density lipoprotein, which is known as bad cholesterol. LDL is bad because
an build up within the walls of your blood vessels and cause atherosclerosis, or plaque build-up, and
ultant narrowing of the passages, which can lead to heart attack or stroke.

ry: Dairy is ok in moderation, if you tolerate dairy.
s would include certain cheeses, milk and yogurt.
stitute frozen yogurt for your ice cream cravings.
RA CREDIT: Greek yogurt tends to be better because
as higher protein and less sugar. Milk from grass-fed
s have Omega 3, 6, 9.

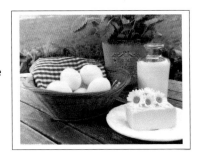

Sugars: Minimize intake of sugars. Particularly avoid high fructose corn syrup. If you are checking nutrition labels, aim to keep the sugar at or below 12g per serving.

Artificial sweeteners are tricky because they can still mimic the body's response to sugar, cause a blood sugar spike and influx of insulin with a resultant crash. In general, avoid artificial sweeteners. However, if you reach for one, keep in mind that Stevia is slightly better than Splenda, and both of these are slightly better than any of the other pink or blue packets you'll see. I'd rather you not add sugar to any food or drink. However, if you are reaching for sugar to put in your coffee, and I absolutely had to give you an answer on which one to choose, pick the one in the brown packet (brown sugar) before any other.

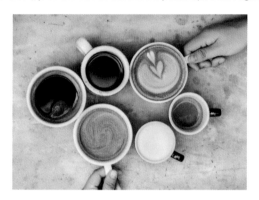

Starches: Minimize intake of potatoes and other starches. These spike blood sugar quickly, similar to highly processed foods. There is a hierarchy if you are going to eat potatoes. Aim for yams or sweet potatoes before your Yukon gold or other white/yellow potato. Corn is a starchy vegetable.

Spices: Ginger root and turmeric are excellent to incorporate in your cooking, as these have natural anti-inflammatory properties and are cardioprotective. Ginger and Turmeric are both excellent for digestive support, boosting your immune system, detoxification and lowering blood sugar. Garlic has a number of health properties, including protecting your heart, helping immunity, and reducing inflammation.

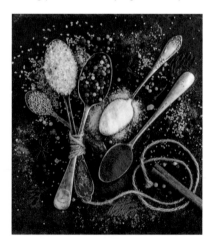

Beverages: Increase water intake. Be sure to drink at least 8oz of water, three times per day.

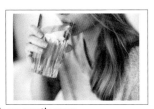

Black coffee is ok, preferably without added cream or sugar. Limit coffee to no more than 16oz per day. Limit or eliminate fruit juices, power drinks and soda as these are often empty calories and high sugar content that will spike your blood sugar levels with little to no nutritional value. The same goes for powdered drinks that you mix with water, which are mostly sugar. Drink alcohol in moderation, not to exceed the equivalent of 1 serving (5 oz) of wine in a 24-hour period. Limit alcohol to no more than four servings per week. Red wine is better than other types of wine due to the resveratrol content, which acts as an antioxidant and AMPK-activator. Keep in mind that most red wine only has a very small percentage of resveratrol, so it's not enough to make a considerable difference in AMPK. Limit consumption of beer and spirits.

If all of this gets confusing, try to remember that your plate should resemble a rainbow: orange, yellow, green and red colors. Typically this is a good indicator that you are getting the fiber, micronutrients and vitamins your body needs in a balanced way.

EXTRA CREDIT / SUPERFOOD SUMMARY: almonds, avocados, spinach, kale, tomatoes, Brussels sprouts, salmon, blueberries, blackberries, açai berry, goji berry, pomegranate, raspberries, flaxseed, chia seed, quinoa, amaranth, milk or butter from grass-fed cows, Greek yogurt.

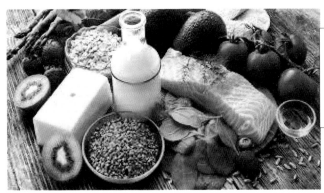

Please see our Cookbook recommendations for more info on RECIPES!

Healthy Splurge and/or Snack Options

Let's be real. We all have moments of weakness. Whether that be a sweet tooth, savory urge or other craving, here are some options to have on hand:

-Guilt-free beverages: Polar seltzer, Spindrift sparkling water, LaCroix sparkling water
-Dark chocolate (the higher the Cacao level the better)
-Frozen yogurt
-Peanut butter with apple slices, brown rice cakes or celery
-Mozzarella cheese sticks
-Hummus with whole wheat pita, wheat thins, baby carrots, cucumber slices, or bell pepper
-Mixed nuts
-Avocado or fresh guacamole
-Olives
-Pistachios
-Hard-boiled egg
-Whole wheat tortilla, black beans, and avocado
-Brown rice bowl with chicken and veggies
-Check the grocery's frozen aisle for organic brown rice, microwave and ready in just a few minutes

Remember your portion sizes!

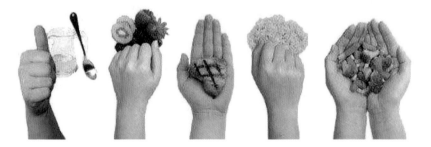

Cookbook Recommendations

- Paleo – Civilized Caveman Cookbooks or The Paleo Kitchen by George Bryant
- Mediterranean – The Complete Mediterranean Cookbook by America's Test Kitchen
- Vegetarian – Clean Eats by Alejandro Junger
- Vegan – Frugal Vegan by Katie Koteen & Kate Kasbee

xercise

0 minutes of cardiovascular exercise *at least* 3 times per week is the minimum recommendation. This eans any type of exercise that gets your heart rate up, for approximately 30 minutes. More frequent xercise is even better.

IIT type of cardiovascular exercise is best. HIIT stands for High Intensity Interval Training. This type of xercise incorporates resistance and/or weight training along with cardiovascular exercise. It is the rfect combination of exercises to ramp up your AMPK activation and activate your metabolism to help urn fat the most effectively. The fact that most HIIT courses tend to be offered as classes is also nice, cause the accountability and support group type of environment is best to keep you motivated.

y type of exercise is good exercise. Make it fun by doing things you naturally enjoy, whether that be king, biking, climbing, rowing, kayaking, swimming, power-walking or dancing. The opportunities are dless, and incorporating exercise in an enjoyable way helps to stimulate the reward center in the ain so that you'll want to keep doing it! Make a playlist of music you enjoy to help pass the time and t you more engaged. Get a workout buddy to help keep you accountable.

HOLE BODY BENEFITS TO EXERCISE: increase serotonin and endorphin levels (feel happier), improve ep, improve cardiovascular system, increase muscle mass and boost basal metabolic rate (burn more ories at rest), increase quality of life and longevity, improve heart and brain function, improve mory, and so much more!

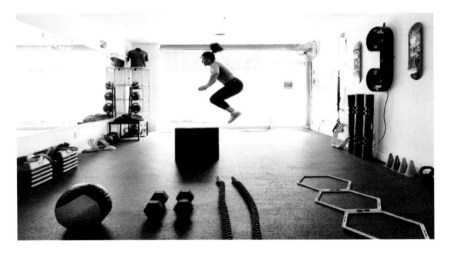

How to Avoid Common Pitfalls

1. Don't let yourself get too hungry = hangry
    - This can cause you to:
      - Overeat and be less mindful about food
      - Have blood sugar spike and resultant crash, which results in worse metabolic function
    - Instead, try to:
      - Keep healthy snacks around, pack your lunch, don't go grocery shopping when you are starving
2. If you're looking for an app to track/monitor calories, we recommend the 'MyFitnessPal' app
3. Aim for smaller portion sizes, push away from the table to allow yourself time to realize you are full.
4. Find an accountability partner: whether that be a friend, a spouse, a relative, or even a Facebook Group where you can connect with others going through similar challenges, to help motivate and encourage you.
    *If you'd like a recommendation, search for the "Metabolic Syndrome Support Group" on Facebook.
5. Decrease stress. Stress increases cortisol, cortisol spikes your blood sugar and decreases your immune system. Find ways to hack stress. Consider meditating, even if only 5-10 minutes per day. Sometimes this can be enough to re-set the neurotransmitters in your brain and result in: decreased stress, decreased cortisol levels, decreased inflammation, improved coping mechanisms and improved creative thinking.
6. Focus on healthy mind, body and spirit. If spirituality is something you with which you identify, incorporate that to further boost your progress and healing process.
7. Realize that YOU can do anything you put your mind to. You are more powerful and capable than your realize. You have control over your life. Focus on small, attainable goals, to avoid getting overwhelmed.
8. Work on having a healthy, positive relationship with food. Avoid using food as a coping mechanism for your feelings, whether that be stress, anger, fear, sadness, reward, or punishment. Take back-up measures to ensure you set yourself up for success.
9. Break old habits and establish new habits. A habit is something that you do because you're used to doing it. Once you replace a bad habit with a good one, and practice that new good ritual daily for a few weeks, surprise! You have a new, fantastic habit.
10. Quality and quantity of **sleep**. Sleep is listed last here, but is certainly not least. In fact, sleep is probably one of the most important factors to your health. Consistently getting less than hours of sleep per night can cause increased levels of cortisol. Sleep deprivation mimics the stress response in your body, and resultant cortisol can accelerate metabolic dysfunction along with a decrease in cognitive functioning. Aim to get 7-9 hours of sleep per night.

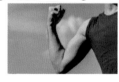

14

What Are Some Prescription Medications that Treat Metabolic Syndrome?

Your doctor may have talked to you about Metabolic Syndrome. What unfortunately all too often can happen is that you are given the diagnosis, but not much education about what it is or what to do next. Relying on Dr. Google can lead to a lot of scattered mis-information.

Some prescriptions that may be associated with Metabolic Syndrome include, but are not limited to:

Blood sugar
Metformin (Glucophage), Sitagliptin (Januvia), Onglyza, Amaryl (Glimepiride), Janumet, Glipizide, Insulin

Blood pressure
Lisinopril, Losartan, Valsartan, Hydrochlorothiazide, Amlodipine, Nifedipine, Coreg, Metoprolol, Atenolol

Cholesterol
Simvastatin, Atorvastatin, Crestor, Lipitor, Zocor, Niacin, Tricor, Zetia, Vytorin

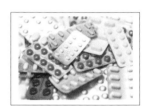

Before you know it, you may find that you are on a bunch of different medications, without fully understanding why you're taking them or what the medicines are doing to your body. Multi-pharmacy can be overwhelming to you and your body, and often there can be medication side-effects.

What Are Some Natural Supplements that Can Help?

- **BestFormin** – all natural herbal combination of Berberine, Green Tea Extract, Garcinia Cambogia
- Alpha Lipoic Acid
- Chromium Picolinate
- Cinnamon

Activates AMPK!

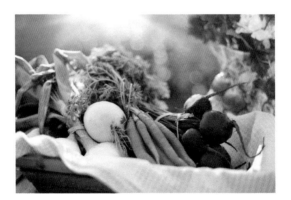

What Is AMPK and Why Do I Want It to Be Activated?

AMPK stands for AMP-activated protein kinase. It is an enzyme in your body that serves a crucial role in regulating your metabolism. It is so important, in fact, that it acts as the "master-regulating switch." When AMPK is activated, it stimulates your body's process to generate energy. In return, your metabolism speeds up and your body burns fat. We all have AMPK in every cell in our body. The problem is, sometimes it is not fully activated.

Vigorous exercise can activate AMPK. Also, by eating a healthy, calorie-controlled diet with intermittent periods of fasting, you can jump-start your AMPK activity.

Scientific studies show that those with Type 2 Diabetes, Pre-Diabetes, and Metabolic Syndrome struggle with largely inactive AMPK. The reason why Metformin is one of the first-line agents for Type 2 Diabetic is because Metformin is an AMPK-activator.

<u>What if you want to find natural ways to activate AMPK?</u>

Many people want a more natural approach to get in shape, successfully improve their stagnant metabolic process, and potentially avoid multiple costly prescriptions. The good news is that there are several natural ways to activate AMPK:

1. **Berberine** is an alkaloid similar to Turmeric, extracted from various plants (i.e. Berberis, tree turmeric goldenseal, yellow root and Oregon grape). Studies show that Berberine is a top-tier natural agent to activate AMPK and rivals the efficacy of Metformin in clinical studies[4,5]. Berberine has myriad additional health benefits, including but not limited to: improved blood sugar & cholesterol, protection of the endothelial lining (benefits for blood pressure), improved gut microbiome, enhanced immune system, and even anti-cancer properties. Berberine has been used for centuries in traditional Chinese and Ayurvedic medicine.

2. **Resveratrol** is a natural phenol that can be found in certain red grapes and red wine, as well as a number of berries including blueberries, raspberries, mulberries and cranberries.

3. **Green tea** and **coffee bean extract**, helps promote weight loss and reduce blood pressure in people with hypertension.

4. **Quercetin** is a flavonoid, which is found in many plants and foods, such as red wine, onions, green tea, apples, berries, Ginkgo biloba, St. John's wort, American elder, and Buckwheat tea.

5. **Genistein** is a phytoestrogen found in a number of plants such as soybeans.

<u>BestFormin</u> is a natural supplement that incorporates Berberine and green tea to activate AMPK, plus Garcinia Cambogia fruit extract to reduce cravings, with the benefit of decreased lipogenesis (fat synthesis) at the cellular level. This unique, high-quality natural remedy helps achieve optimal results.

In summary, studies suggest that AMPK-activators are a natural way to help prevent obesity and Type Diabetes, reduce body weight and lipid levels, and improve insulin sensitivity.

What Is Berberine, and Why Should I Take It?

What Is Berberine

Berberine is a yellow-colored alkaloid compound which is extracted from various plants. Some of the plants include Berberis, tree turmeric, goldenseal, yellow root and Oregon grape. Berberine has been used for centuries in traditional Chinese medicine and Ayurvedic medicine.

What Is Berberine Used For?

Berberine is a metabolic activator at the mitochondrial level.

It affects your body at the molecular level and functions inside cells, having many benefits for various health issues. One of the most important functions of Berberine is its ability to activate AMPK. AMPK optimizes cell metabolism.

Berberine benefits your health in numerous ways. Most commonly, it is used as a natural way to support healthy blood sugar levels. This means that it is an excellent supplement for healthy weight loss, because healthy and stable blood sugar levels are essential for weight loss, and maintaining healthy weight. It also supports your immune system, cardiovascular health, and gut health. It is been shown by multiple scientific studies to promote healthy cholesterol and lipid levels[3,4]. It has been shown to support the gut microbiome[3,4] (the population of *good* bacteria in our gut).

Head-to-head studies comparing Berberine and Metformin show similar achievements with regard to increased hemoglobin A1C levels at the 3- and 6-month markers[5]. This means that Berberine is as good as Metformin with regard to lowering blood sugar levels, and Berberine surpasses Metformin with regard to cholesterol-lowering, among many other benefits.

Berberine helps with blood sugar levels, cholesterol, gut health: microbiome, anti-inflammatory, anti-cancer, immune system, cholesterol, targeted fat loss (weight loss), cardiovascular health and longevity.†

BestFormin is a natural dietary supplement that incorporates **Berberine**, **Green Tea Extract** and **Garcinia Cambogia** with the goal of supporting those with Metabolic Syndrome. If used in conjunction with a healthy diet and exercise, it can enhance your results and help you see results faster.
Other potential advantage: it may help reduce the number of other supplements or medications you're taking†. Please consult your doctor. Visit this website for more information: www.dochox.com

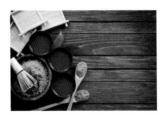

Summary

Metabolic Syndrome is an increasing problem. 1 out of 3 Americans have Metabolic Syndrome, and it even affects 1 out of 5 children and adolescents. The statistics increase to a dramatic 50% of those over age 60[1].

Those with Metabolic Syndrome are at increased risk for Type 2 Diabetes, heart disease and stroke. Lifestyle changes can potentially reverse this diagnosis.

We've discussed the importance of a calorie-controlled diet, with nutrient-rich foods to fuel and nourish your body, along with exercise methods to help you be successful. We have provided you options for dietary supplementation to perfectly complement your diet and exercise routine.

Having a healthy relationship with food is important. If you struggle with an unhealthy relationship with food like binging, purging, or restriction, or if you struggle with anxiety or depression, know that you are not alone, and please reach out for help. Realize that your support group is bigger than you can imagine. We are here for you, and if you need help, please let us or your doctor know so that we can be a team and make progress together. My goal is to provide helpful information, empower you, and support you along your journey to better health. I hope the information in this book will add value to your life.

If you have interest, please follow us on social media platforms. Your questions are welcome and encouraged. Be sure to join the **Metabolic Syndrome Support Group** Facebook Page! There, you'll find recipes, exercise techniques, and motivational mindset tools.

Thanks for reading!

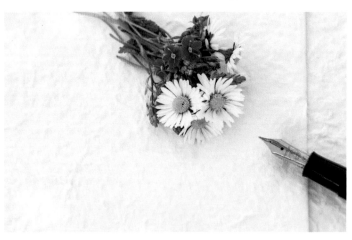

Instagram   Facebook   FB - Support Group   Twitter   Email

APPENDIX

More Information

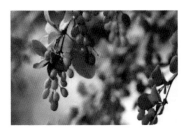

BERBERINE HCL

Berberine is a highly researched alkaloid extracted from various plants (i.e. Berberis, tree turmeric, Goldenseal, yellow root and Oregon grape), and widely used in botanical medical practice. It has a long history of use in ancient Indian and traditional Chinese medicines, and has been used as a treatment to various ailments for hundreds of years.

SOME BENEFITS OF BERBERINE MAY INCLUDE†:

- Improved function at cellular level with regards to optimizing cellular energy and glucose metabolism

- Stabilized blood sugar levels

- Decreased glycogen synthesis, increased glucose uptake and utilization

- Inhibited fatty acid and cholesterol synthesis

- Weight loss particularly in the midsection (decrease in belly fat)

- Anti-inflammatory effects

- Improved intestinal health

- Improved cholesterol levels

- Improved heart health

- Improved immune system via optimization of microbiome

- Antibacterial and anti-yeast properties

- Improved mood and gentle boost in energy

- Protective to the neurologic system

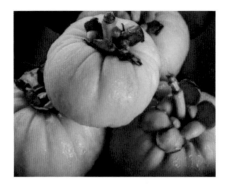

GARCINIA CAMBOGIA

Garcinia Cambogia is a fruit extract that acts as a natural fat burner and appetite suppressant, making weight loss much easier to accomplish†.

SOME BENEFITS OF GARCINIA CAMBOGIA MAY INCLUDE†:

- Decreased lipogenesis (fat synthesis)

- Improved ability to lose weight due to natural appetite suppression and thermogenesis (body ability to burn calories faster)

- Boosted metabolism

- Lowered cholesterol and blood pressure

- Improved heart health

- Improved digestion

- Strengthened immune system due to it being rich in Vitamin C and anti-oxidant properties

- Decreased cellular damage

- Protection to stomach against ulcers

- Improved mental alertness and serotonin levels

- Enhanced energy

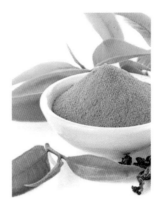

GREEN TEA LEAF EXTRACT

SOME BENEFITS OF GREEN TEA LEAF EXTRACT MAY INCLUDE†:

- Improved stamina and immunity
- Delayed signs and symptoms of aging
- Improved blood circulation and blood pressure
- Toned muscle and skin
- Improved cholesterol
- Antioxidant and detoxification properties
- Decreased stress
- Reduced body fat
- Improved mood
- Optimized brain activity and memory

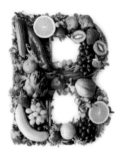

B VITAMINS

Vitamin B6, B7 (Biotin), and B12

These B vitamins help the body as an enzyme cofactor. The B vitamins found in the BestFormin formula, have been shown to have a synergistic effect of the blood sugar-controlling properties, helping to even out blood glucose levels naturally†.

SOME BENEFITS OF THESE B-VITAMINS MAY INCLUDE†:

- Optimized functioning of immune system

- Protection of the central nervous system

- Increased energy and stamina

- Improved heart health

- Balanced hormones and mood

- Regulated blood sugar

- Enhanced weight loss and metabolism

- Improved cholesterol

- Strengthened skin, hair and nails

- Growth and maintenance of muscle tissue

- Improved mood

- Optimized brain activity and memory

- Improved mental clarity

- Improved sleep

†Disclaimer: These statements have not been evaluated by the Food and Drug Administration. These products are not intended diagnose, treat, cure or prevent any disease. Product results may vary from person to person

References

Prevalence of the Metabolic Syndrome in the United States, 2003-2012. Maria Aguilar, MD1; Taft ꞏuket, MD2; Sharon Torres, PA2; et al. *JAMA*. 2015;313(19):1973-1974. doi:10.1001/jama.2015.4260. tps://jamanetwork.com/journals/jama/fullarticle/2293286

UpToDate. The Metabolic Syndrome (insulin resistance syndrome or syndrome X). UpToDate. James B eigs, MD. 2019 Jan 15. https://www.uptodate.com/contents/the-metabolic-syndrome-insulin-sistance-syndrome-or-syndrome-ꞏsearch=metabolic%20syndrome&source=search_result&selectedTitle=1~150&usage_type=default&di ꞏlay_rank=1

Berberine – A Powerful Supplement with Many Benefits. Kris Gunnars, BSc. 2017 Jan 14. tps://www.healthline.com/nutrition/berberine-powerful-supplement#section3

Clinical Applications for Berberine: Potential therapeutic applications in metabolic syndrome, type 2 ꞏbetes, and dyslipidemia. Jacob Schor, ND, FABNO. December 2012 Vol. 4 Issue 12. tps://www.naturalmedicinejournal.com/journal/2012-12/clinical-applications-berberine

Efficacy of berberine in patients with type 2 diabetes mellitus. Yin J1, Xing H, Ye J. *Metabolism*. 2008 ꞏay;57(5):712-7. https://www.ncbi.nlm.nih.gov/pubmed/18442638

Definitions of the metabolic syndrome. UpToDate. James B Meigs, MD. 2019 Jan 15. ꞏps://www.uptodate.com/contents/image?csi=5ecd2a7d-58a5-4bf7-9692-ꞏ5807664c48&source=contentShare&imageKey=ENDO%2F53446

Alberti KG, Eckel RH, Grundy SM, et al. Harmonizing the metabolic syndrome: a joint interim ꞏtement of the International Diabetes Federation Task Force on Epidemiology and Prevention; ꞏtional Heart, Lung, and Blood Institute; American Heart Association; World Heart Federation; ꞏernational Atherosclerosis Society; and International Association for the Study of Obesity. Circulation ꞏ9; 120:1640.

Meigs J. Metabolic syndrome and risk for type 2 diabetes. *Expert Rev Endocrin Metab 2006*; 1:57. ꞏle 1. Updated data from the International Diabetes Federation, 2006.

Table 1: Definitions of the metabolic syndrome[6,7,8]

NCEP: National Cholesterol Education Program; IDF: International Diabetes Federation; WHO: World Health Organization; AACE: American Association of Clinical Endocrinologists; HDL: high density lipoprotein; BMI: body mass index.

* Most commonly agreed upon criteria for metabolic syndrome (any three of five risk factors).

Parameters	NCEP ATP3 2005*	IDF 2006	WHO 1999	AACE 2003
Required		Waist ≥94 cm (men) or ≥80 cm (women)¶	Insulin resistance in top 25%⁰; glucose ≥6.1 mmol/L (110 mg/dL); 2-hour glucose ≥7.8 mmol/L (140 mg/dL)	High risk of insulin resistance⁺ or BMI ≥25 kg/m² or waist ≥102 cm (men) or ≥88 cm (women)
Number of abnormalities	≥3 of:	And ≥2 of:	And ≥2 of:	And ≥2 of:
Glucose	≥5.6 mmol/L (100 mg/dL) or drug treatment for elevated blood glucose	≥5.6 mmol/L (100 mg/dL) or diagnosed diabetes		≥6.1 mmol/L (110 mg/dL); ≥2 hour glucose 7.8 mmol/L (140 mg/dL)
HDL cholesterol	<1.0 mmol/L (40 mg/dL) (men); <1.3 mmol/L (50 mg/dL) (women) or drug treatment for low HDL cholesterol¹	<1.0 mmol/L (40 mg/dL) (men); <1.3 mmol/L (50 mg/dL) (women) or drug treatment for low HDL cholesterol	<0.9 mmol/L (35 mg/dL) (men); <1.0 mmol/L (40 mg/dL) (women)	<1.0 mmol/L (40 mg/dL) (men); <1.3 mmol/L (50 mg/dL) (women)
Triglycerides	≥1.7 mmol/L (150 mg/dL) or drug treatment for elevated triglycerides¹	≥1.7 mmol/L (150 mg/dL) or drug treatment for high triglycerides	or ≥1.7 mmol/L (150 mg/dL)	≥1.7 mmol/L (150 mg/dL)
Obesity	Waist ≥102 cm (men) or ≥88 cm (women)⁸		Waist/hip ratio >0.9 (men) or >0.85 (women) or BMI ≥30 kg/m²	
Hypertension	≥130/85 mmHg or drug treatment for hypertension	≥130/85 mmHg or drug treatment for hypertension	≥140/90 mmHg	≥130/85 mmHg

Printed by Amazon Italia Logistica S.r.l.
Torrazza Piemonte (TO), Italy

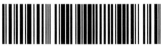

12832964R00016